Kamel Bengayed

The basics of maternal-fetal anesthesia and resuscitation

Kamel Bengayed

The basics of maternal-fetal anesthesia and resuscitation

for midwives

ScienciaScripts

Cover image: www.ingimage.com

This book is a translation from the original published under ISBN 978-620-6-71067-7.

Publisher:
Sciencia Scripts
is a trademark of
Dodo Books Indian Ocean Ltd. and OmniScriptum S.R.L publishing group

120 High Road, East Finchley, London, N2 9ED, United Kingdom
Str. Armeneasca 28/1, office 1, Chisinau MD-2012, Republic of Moldova, Europe
Printed at: see last page
ISBN: 978-620-8-08540-7

Table of contents

Management of post-partum haemorrhage

Theoretical objectives :

1. Detect risk factors for postpartum haemorrhage (PPH).

2. Diagnose the various causes of postpartum haemorrhage.

3. Describe the algorithm for the initial management of PPH.

1. Definition of postpartum haemorrhage (PPH) :

PPH is a serious obstetric complication defined as excessive blood loss following childbirth. The definition threshold varies according to the mode of delivery:

- Lower tract: Blood loss greater than 500 ml
- Caesarean section: Blood loss greater than 1000 ml

It is important to note that quantifying blood loss can be difficult and is often underestimated. Thus, rigorous clinical assessment and careful monitoring of vital signs are crucial in identifying PPH.

PPH is a potentially fatal obstetric emergency. It can lead to hypovolaemic shock, renal failure or even multiple organ failure and, in extreme cases, maternal death. Rapid and effective management is therefore essential to minimise the risks and preserve maternal health.

2. Etiologies of PPH :

There are many causes of PPH, which can be classified according to the "4T" model:

Tonus: Uterine atony is the most common cause of PPH. It is characterised by the inability of the uterus to contract effectively after childbirth, which impairs haemostasis at the placental site. Several factors can lead to uterine atony, including an over-distended uterus (multiple pregnancy, hydramnios), prolonged labour, excessive use of oxytocin, general anaesthesia and infections.

Tissue: Retention of placental fragments or membranes in the uterus can prevent proper uterine dynamics and subsequently cause persistent haemorrhage. Careful examination of the placenta after delivery is crucial to identify any abnormalities.

Trauma: Injuries to the reproductive tract, such as tears to the cervix, vagina, uterus or pelvic blood vessels, can cause severe bleeding. These injuries can occur during a difficult delivery, an instrumental extraction (forceps, suction cup) or a caesarean section.

Thrombin: Coagulation disorders, whether pre-existing (von Willebrand disease, haemophilia) or acquired (disseminated intravascular coagulation, HELLP syndrome), can interfere with the formation of blood clots and lead to excessive bleeding.

3. Risk factors :

Several factors can increase the risk of developing PPH:

History of PPH: A history of PPH is a major risk factor for haemorrhage in subsequent deliveries.

Hypertensive uterus: An over-distended uterus, for example in the case of multiple pregnancy, hydramnios or foetal macrosomia, is more likely to be atonic after childbirth.

Prolonged labour or instrumental delivery: Prolonged labour can exhaust the uterine muscle and increase the risk of atony. Instrumental deliveries (forceps, vacuum) increase the risk of damage to the genital tract.

Placental abnormalities: Placenta previa (placenta implanted low in the uterus) and placental abruption (premature separation of the placenta) are associated with an increased risk of PPH.

Coagulation disorders: Coagulation disorders, whether known or undiagnosed, can complicate haemostasis and increase the risk of haemorrhage.

Obesity: Obesity is associated with an increased risk of obstetric complications, including PPH.

Primiparity: Women giving birth for the first time have a slightly higher risk of PPH.

4. Early diagnosis of PPH :

Vigilance and rigorous clinical assessment are essential if PPH is to be rapidly identified and appropriate management put in place.

Here are the key elements of surveillance:

Assessment of blood loss: Quantifying blood loss is essential for assessing the severity of the haemorrhage. Weighing the compresses and measuring the volume of blood in the drains provides a more accurate estimate than simple observation.

Monitoring vital signs: Close monitoring of vital signs (pulse, blood pressure) can detect the first signs of hypovolaemic shock, especially tachycardia, which is the earliest sign.

Palpation of the uterus: Palpation of the abdomen is used to assess uterine tone. A soft, slack uterus suggests atony.

Examination of the placenta: Careful examination of the placenta after delivery ensures its integrity and detects any abnormalities or retained fragments.

5. Management of PPH :

The management of PPH follows a precise algorithm aimed at controlling bleeding, restoring blood volume and identifying and treating the underlying cause. The speed and coordination of the medical team are crucial.

Call for help: In the event of suspected or confirmed PPH, it is essential to call for help immediately. This involves mobilising the medical team (obstetrician, anaesthetist, midwife, nurse, laboratory staff) and preparing the necessary equipment (uterotonics, vascular filling fluids, blood products).

Uterine massage and administration of uterotonics: External uterine massage aims to stimulate uterine contractions and promote haemostasis. Uterotonics, such as oxytocin, are administered to reinforce uterine contractions.

Vascular filling: The aim of vascular filling is to restore circulating blood volume and prevent hypovolaemic shock. Crystalloids (lactated Ringer's, isotonic saline) and macromolecules (albumin, etc.) may be used.

Finding the cause and treating the aetiology: Once the haemorrhage is under control, it is important to identify the underlying cause and treat it. Depending on the cause, this may involve:

Suturing lesions: In the case of genital tract tears, surgical suturing is necessary to stop the bleeding.

Evacuating a haematoma: If a haematoma has formed, it may need to be evacuated.

Uterine exploration: If retained placental fragments or membranes are suspected, manual exploration of the uterus can be carried out under anaesthetic.

Arterial embolisation: In some cases, a radiological technique called arterial embolisation can be used to block the blood vessels that are maintaining the haemorrhage.

Hysterectomy: In cases of uncontrollable PPH, a hysterectomy may be necessary as a last resort to save the mother's life.

Blood transfusion: If blood loss is significant, the administration of blood products or other blood derivatives may be necessary to restore haemostasis and the oxygen-carrying capacity of the blood.

Close monitoring: Close monitoring of vital parameters (pulse, blood pressure, oxygen saturation), bleeding and diuresis is essential to assess response to treatment and detect any complications.

6. Key Concepts :

To complete your understanding of the management of PPH, it is important to take a closer look at certain key concepts:

a. Assessment of blood volume and shock :

Signs and symptoms of hypovolaemic shock: Monitoring vital signs is crucial for early detection of hypovolaemic shock. Signs include tachycardia, hypotension, decreased oxygen saturation, skin pallor, oliguria (decreased urine volume), agitation and confusion.

Advanced haemodynamic monitoring: In severe cases, invasive haemodynamic monitoring may be necessary to accurately assess blood volume status and guide fluid resuscitation.

Shock indices: Indices such as the Shock Index (SI = heart rate / systolic blood pressure) and the Modified Shock Index (MSI = heart rate / mean arterial pressure) can help assess the severity of shock and guide treatment decisions.

b. Coagulation management :

Assessment of coagulation status: Laboratory tests such as prothrombin time (PT), activated partial thromboplastin time (APTT) and platelet count are used to assess coagulation function.

Blood products: In the event of coagulation disorders or massive haemorrhage, a transfusion of blood products (packed red blood cells, fresh frozen plasma, platelets) may be necessary.

Haemostatic drugs: Drugs such as tranexamic acid can be used to boost coagulation and reduce blood loss.

c. Post-HPP care :

Ongoing monitoring: Patients with PPH require close monitoring for several hours or days after the event. This includes monitoring vital signs, bleeding, diuresis, neurological status and pain.

Pain management: Post-partum pain can be exacerbated by PPH and its treatment. Adequate analgesia is essential for the patient's comfort and well-being.

Psychological support: PPH can be a traumatic experience for women and their families. Psychological support is important to help manage post-traumatic stress and the emotions associated with the event.

d. Multidisciplinary aspects :

Collaboration with other healthcare professionals: The management of PPH requires close collaboration between midwives, obstetricians, anaesthetists, nurses and other healthcare professionals.

Transfer to a specialist centre: In complex or severe cases, transfer to a specialist centre with resources and expertise in obstetric intensive care may be necessary.

e. Prevention of PPH :

Identifying patients at risk: Assessing risk factors before delivery helps to identify women at risk of PPH and to implement preventive measures.

Active management of the third stage of labour: Administration of oxytocin after delivery of the baby and controlled traction of the umbilical cord can reduce the risk of PPH.

Management of labour and delivery: Careful monitoring of labour and delivery, and early intervention in the event of complications, can minimise the risk of PPH.

f. Research and Innovation :

New technologies: Uterine compression devices and intrauterine balloons are being developed to improve the management of PPH.

New haemostatic drugs: Ongoing research into haemostatic drugs is aimed at finding more effective and safer options for controlling bleeding.

Improving management protocols: Clinical studies and regular audits of practices are needed to improve management protocols and optimise patient outcomes.

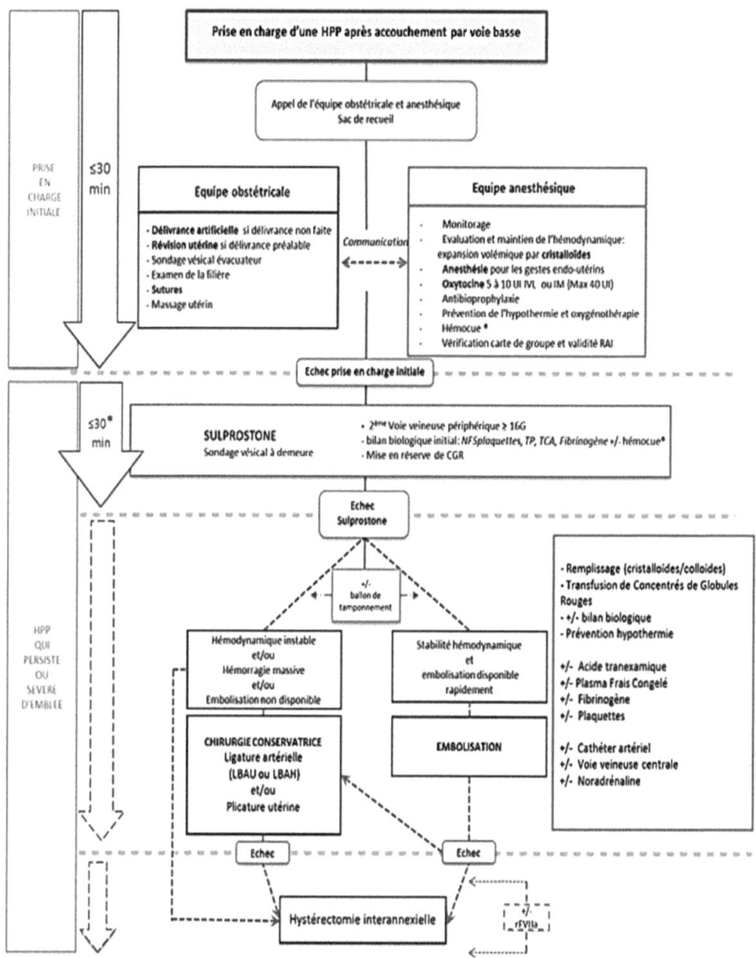

Figure 1: Decision-making algorithm for PPH after vaginal delivery

https://sfar.org/prise-en-charge-de-lhemorragie-du-post-partum/

g. Ethics and Psychological Aspects :

Informed consent: Patients must be informed of the risks and benefits of the different PPH treatment options before making informed decisions.

Respect for the patient's autonomy : The patient's choices and preferences must be respected as far as possible.

Emotional support: Midwives must be sensitive to the emotional needs of patients and their families and offer them appropriate support and information.

Managing stress and anxiety: PPH can be a stressful experience for midwives. It is important to develop strategies for managing stress and anxiety in order to maintain an optimal level of performance in an emergency situation.

In conclusion, the management of PPH requires a thorough knowledge of the causes, risk factors, treatment options and multidisciplinary aspects of this obstetric emergency. As future midwives, it is essential that you familiarise yourself with the latest recommendations and develop the skills needed to effectively manage patients with PPH, while offering them empathetic and respectful support.

7. Conclusion

PPH is a serious obstetric emergency requiring rapid and effective management. Early recognition of the risk factors and signs of PPH, and appropriate management according to the established algorithm, are essential to improve the maternal prognosis and prevent potentially fatal complications.

As midwives, you play a crucial role in the prevention, early diagnosis and initial management of PPH. Your clinical expertise and ability to react quickly in emergency situations can save lives.

References

1. Royal College of Obstetricians and Gynaecologists. Prevention and management of postpartum haemorrhage. Green-top Guideline No. 52. London: RCOG; 2016.

This comprehensive guide from the RCOG provides evidence-based recommendations for the prevention and management of PPH, covering risk assessment, preventive measures, active management protocols for the third stage of labour, pharmacological and surgical treatment options, and post-PPH care.

2. World Health Organization. WHO recommendations for the prevention and treatment of postpartum haemorrhage. Geneva: WHO; 2012.

This WHO document provides global recommendations for the prevention and treatment of PPH, with a focus on low-resource settings. It covers the use of uterotonics, active management of the third stage of labour, treatment of uterine atony and management of severe cases.

3. American College of Obstetricians and Gynecologists. ACOG Practice Bulletin No. 183: Postpartum hemorrhage. Obstet Gynecol. 2017;130(4):e168-e186.

This ACOG practice bulletin provides evidence-based guidelines for the management of PPH, including assessment, initial treatment, cause-specific treatment options, and post-PPH care.

4. Mousa HA, Alfirevic Z. Treatment for primary postpartum haemorrhage. Cochrane Database Syst Rev. 2017;9:CD003249.

This Cochrane review analyses the available evidence on the various treatments for primary HPP, comparing their efficacy and adverse effects. It provides valuable information to guide therapeutic decisions.

5. Sentilhes L, Vayssière C, Deneux-Tharaux C, et al. Postpartum hemorrhage: guidelines for clinical practice from the French College of Gynaecologists and Obstetricians (CNGOF). Eur J Obstet Gynecol Reprod Biol. 2016;207:143-156.

These CNGOF guidelines provide a comprehensive overview of the management of PPH, covering prevention, diagnosis, different treatment options and specific aspects of management, such as blood transfusion and intensive care.

Questions

1. What are the main differences in the definition of PPH depending on the mode of delivery (vaginal delivery vs caesarean section)?

Answer: PPH is defined as blood loss of more than 500 ml after vaginal delivery and more than 1000 ml after caesarean section.

2. Explain why uterine atony is the most common cause of PPH.

Answer: Uterine atony is the inability of the uterus to contract effectively after childbirth, which prevents haemostasis at the placental site and leads to haemorrhage.

3. Describe the key steps in clinical assessment for early detection of PPH.

Answer: The clinical assessment of PPH includes evaluation of blood loss (weighing of compresses, measurement of volume in drains), monitoring of vital signs (pulse, blood pressure), palpation of the uterus to assess tone and examination of the placenta to check its integrity.

4. Why does the management of PPH require rapid, coordinated action?

Answer: PPH is a life-threatening emergency. Rapid, coordinated action is essential to control the bleeding, prevent shock and improve the mother's chances of survival.

5. Explain why identifying the underlying cause of PPH is important for treatment.

Answer: Identifying the cause allows specific treatment to be adapted to the situation, which increases the chances of success and reduces the risk of complications.

Multidisciplinary management of pre-eclampsia

Learning objectives :

1. Define gestational hypertension, pre-eclampsia and associated convulsions.

2. Identify the signs of severity and seriousness in a patient with pre-eclampsia.

3. Recognise the criteria for obstetric intervention, use of magnesium sulphate and antihypertensive treatments.

4. Understanding the anaesthetic management of a parturient with pre-eclampsia.

5. Explain the anaesthetic management of a parturient with eclampsia.

1. Conceptual framework :

Gestational hypertension: Increase in blood pressure during pregnancy, without additional signs of placental dysfunction. A distinction is made between chronic (present before pregnancy) and gestational (appearing after 20 weeks) forms.

Pre-eclampsia: Gestational hypertension accompanied by proteinuria (≥ 300mg/24h) or organ dysfunction (headache, visual disturbances, abdominal pain, nausea/vomiting, oliguria, liver abnormalities, thrombocytopenia) after 20 weeks' gestation.

Eclampsia: generalised convulsive seizures or unexplained coma in a woman suffering from pre-eclampsia: this is a medical emergency with a life-threatening impact on the mother and foetus.

2. Awareness-raising and training :

It is important to inform pregnant women and professionals about the signs and symptoms of pre-eclampsia. It is also important to involve pregnant women in regular prenatal check-ups to monitor blood pressure and detect abnormalities.

3. Prediction and prevention :

It is important to identify the risk factors (previous history, maternal pathologies, multiple pregnancies, etc.) and to suggest preventive measures (e.g. low-dose aspirin).

4. Management of pre-eclampsia

a. Coordinated care network :

Primary and secondary care healthcare professionals must work together to ensure optimal follow-up and rapid intervention where necessary.

b. Pre-hospital and inter-hospital care :

Care must be organised before any transfer. To avoid complications during this phase, the severity of the situation needs to be properly assessed on the basis of blood pressure, proteinuria, clinical signs and biological tests. Blood pressure and foetal well-being need to be monitored and ultrasound scans performed, so that a decision can be taken on transfer to a suitable facility if necessary.

c. Hospital treatment :

As soon as the patient is admitted to the maternity ward, the patient's history and functional and physical signs should be checked (BP measurement + urine dipstick to look for proteinuria) and the necessary biological tests should be ordered (haemoglobin, platelets, creatininemia, transaminases + 24-hour proteinuria), as well as continuous maternal and foetal monitoring.

Antihypertensive treatment to control blood pressure and magnesium sulphate to prevent convulsions should be indicated as recommended, following the advice of the anaesthetist-resuscitator.

It is necessary to assess foetal maturity and decide on extraction depending on the situation.

d. Criteria for termination of pregnancy :

The decision to extract the foetus depends on :

- The presence or absence of signs of seriousness.

- The term of pregnancy and foetal maturity.
- Foetal well-being.

5. Complication management

Convulsions: Management must be urgent, with protection of the airways and administration of oxygen, and quickly ensure that the vascular approach is patent for administration of magnesium sulphate IVD if the patient is convulsing and IVL over 30 minutes if she has returned to her baseline state, and go to the operating theatre for emergency foetal extraction, but at least make sure that a blood test has been sent to the laboratory as a matter of urgency, because having an updated haemoglobin and platelet count back quickly will help with the anaesthetic decision.

Renal impairment: renal function must be monitored (diuresis and creatinine levels) and fluid intake must be optimised (not too much to avoid pulmonary alveolar overload, not too little to avoid hypovolaemia, which can lead to renal failure).

Hepatic impairment: liver function tests must be monitored, at a rate appropriate to the expectant period decided.

Retroplacental haematoma: A premature detachment of the placenta must be sought on ultrasound, especially if there are signs in favour of this, such as foetal distress with high blood pressure and maternal tachycardia, or the presence of maternal conjunctival pallor. Treatment must be urgent: correction of haemostasis problems by transfusion of blood derivatives and the decision to extract the foetus immediately.

6. Anaesthesia in pre-eclampsia :

The choice of anaesthetic technique must be adapted to the clinical and biological situation and to comorbidities.

If the patient has convulsed only once, with a return to normal neurological status, a stable clinical condition and a platelet count acceptable for lumbar puncture, the patient may be given a short course of anaesthesia.

A general anaesthetic with a rapid induction sequence and the addition of remifentanil if blood pressure is high, to avoid a hypertensive peak at the time of intubation.

The risk of difficult intubation is greater in pregnant women than in other populations, especially with the increased pharyngeal oedema in pre-eclampsia patients, and especially if they are already in labour.

On the other hand, pregnant women are considered to have a full stomach, even if they have not eaten anything for 6 hours, but a meal in the last 6 hours increases the risk of inhalation during intubation.

It is therefore crucial to check that there is a functional source of mucus suction during anaesthetic induction.

Care must be taken with intraoperative fluid intake, to avoid inducing PAO through fluid overload, and renal failure through inadequate intake.

The platelet count should be checked and haemostasis monitored (PT, APTT), especially if there is a history of HRP or HELLP syndrome.

7. After pre-eclampsia

Prognosis for children: expectant mothers should be informed of the increased risk of prematurity, growth retardation and possible neonatal complications.

Early post-partum monitoring: the mother-to-be should be informed of the importance of monitoring blood pressure, kidney and liver function, the risk of haemorrhage and thromboembolic complications.

Long-term follow-up: given the increased risk of cardiovascular disease for the mother, she needs to be committed to regular medical check-ups and a healthy lifestyle.

8. Recapitalisation of key concepts :

a. Pathophysiology of pre-eclampsia :

The exact cause remains unknown, but the main hypothesis involves abnormal placental implantation leading to poor vascularisation and placental hypoxia. This triggers a cascade of reactions with the release of anti-angiogenic and inflammatory factors, leading to generalised endothelial dysfunction and hypertension.

b. Risk factors :

Previous history: Preeclampsia in a previous pregnancy, family history of preeclampsia.

Maternal pathologies: chronic hypertension, diabetes, autoimmune diseases (lupus), antiphospholipid syndrome, obesity.

Pregnancy: Multiple pregnancy, molar pregnancy, first child, maternal age < 20 years or > 40 years.

Other: History of thrombosis, thrombophilia, placental anomalies.

c. Classification of severity :

Mild pre-eclampsia: Hypertension and proteinuria without signs of severity.

Severe pre-eclampsia: Severe arterial hypertension, significant proteinuria and/or signs of organ dysfunction (cerebral, hepatic, renal, haematological, pulmonary).

Eclampsia: Convulsions or coma in a woman with pre-eclampsia.

HELLP syndrome: Haemolysis, Elevated liver enzymes, Low platelets (thrombocytopenia).

d. Magnesium sulphate :

Drug of choice for the prevention and treatment of convulsions. Acts by reducing neuronal excitability and relaxing vascular smooth muscle. Monitoring of osteotendinous reflexes and respiratory rate to detect possible intoxication.

e. Antihypertensive treatment :

Objective: to maintain adequate blood pressure in order to prevent maternal and foetal complications. Choice of drug according to clinical situation and co-morbidities. Close monitoring of adverse effects and impact on foetal well-being.

f. Implications for the role of the midwife :

The midwife's role is crucial in the early detection of pre-eclampsia, patient education and monitoring of pregnant women at risk, as well as working closely with doctors to ensure optimal management and appropriate post-partum follow-up.

References

1 Collège National des Gynécologues Obstétriciens Français (CNGOF). Recommendations for clinical practice. 2019.

2 Société Française d'Anesthésie et de Réanimation (SFAR). Recommendations for clinical practice. 2019.

Questions

1. What is the specific sign of pre-eclampsia?

2. What is the treatment of choice for preventing convulsions in pre-eclampsia?

3. What are the main preventive measures for women at high risk of pre-eclampsia?

4. What are the main biological tests carried out to assess the severity of pre-eclampsia?

5. What are the main anaesthetic techniques available for caesarean sections in cases of pre-eclampsia?

6. What are the signs of worsening that a midwife should look out for in a patient hospitalised for pre-eclampsia?

7. What is HELLP syndrome, a possible complication of pre-eclampsia?

8. Why is long-term follow-up important for women with pre-eclampsia?

Answers:

1. Proteinuria: urine examination: urine dipstick

2. Magnesium sulphate

3. Low-dose aspirin and rigorous prenatal monitoring.

4. Blood count, liver function test, kidney function test, proteinuria test.

5. Spinal anaesthesia or general anaesthesia, depending on the clinical situation.

6. Increased blood pressure, persistent headaches, visual disturbances, abdominal pain, oliguria, etc.

7. Haemolysis (destruction of red blood cells), increased liver enzymes and thrombocytopenia (reduced platelets).

8. To monitor their cardiovascular health and prevent possible long-term complications.

Thromboembolic Disease in the Pregnant Woman

Educational objectives :

1. Identify the main risk factors and pathophysiological mechanisms of venous thromboembolism in pregnant women.

2. Identifying deep vein thrombosis in pregnant women.

3. Recognising pulmonary embolism in pregnant women.

4. List the primary prevention measures for venous thromboembolism recommended for pregnant women, according to their level of risk.

1. Introduction

Pregnancy is a physiological state that induces profound changes in a woman's cardiovascular system. These changes, which are essential for the development of the foetus, also increase the risk of thromboembolic disease (TED). TTE includes deep vein thrombosis (DVT) and pulmonary embolism (PE), two potentially serious conditions that can threaten the health of both mother and baby. As a midwife, understanding this risk and knowing how to manage it are crucial to ensuring a safe pregnancy and birth.

2. Pathophysiology: A delicate balance

Pregnancy orchestrates a complex set of haemostatic changes that favour hypercoagulability. This increase in blood clotting capacity is designed to prevent potentially fatal haemorrhage during childbirth.

Hypercoagulability: The increase in coagulation factors, such as fibrinogen and factor VII, and the decrease in natural anticoagulant factors, such as protein S, create an environment conducive to the formation of clots.

Venous stasis: Compression of the inferior vena cava by the pregnant uterus and hormonal changes slow venous return from the lower limbs, encouraging blood stagnation and thrombus formation.

Endothelial damage: Obstetrical trauma, caesarean section and certain underlying pathologies can damage the inner lining of blood vessels, providing an anchor site for clot formation.

3. Risk Factors: A Profile to Monitor

Some pregnant women are at increased risk of VTE. Identifying these factors is essential for individualised preventive management.

Personal or family history of VTE: A personal or family history of VTE considerably increases the risk of recurrence during pregnancy.

Obesity: Excess weight is associated with increased insulin resistance and a pro-inflammatory state, which favours thrombosis.

Advanced maternal age (>35 years): Advanced age correlates with an increased risk of pregnancy complications, including VTE.

Multiple pregnancy: The presence of several foetuses accentuates the physiological changes of pregnancy and increases the risk of VTE.

Prolonged immobilisation: Lack of mobility, whether due to hospitalisation, prolonged bed rest or long journeys, slows venous return and encourages blood stasis.

Caesarean section: Surgery, particularly caesarean section, is associated with an increased risk of VTE due to trauma to the blood vessels and post-operative immobilisation.

Maternal pathologies: Certain medical conditions, such as thrombophilia (genetic predisposition to thrombosis), anti-phospholipid syndrome (autoimmune disease), cancer and autoimmune diseases, significantly increase the risk of VTE.

4. Diagnosis: A Clinical and Instrumental Approach

The diagnosis of VTE is based on a combination of clinical signs and additional tests.

Clinical signs: The clinical signs of DVT and PE are described in the following sections.

Additional tests:

Venous Doppler ultrasonography: This examination enables the veins of the lower limbs to be visualised and the presence of thrombus to be detected.

Thoracic angioscan: This is the gold standard for diagnosing PE. It enables the pulmonary arteries to be visualised and the presence of an embolus to be detected.

D-dimer: These coagulation markers are elevated in cases of thrombosis, but their levels may also be elevated in other situations, such as pregnancy itself, which limits their specificity.

5. Deepening Key Concepts

Thrombophilia: This is a genetic predisposition to thrombosis. The most common thrombophilias are factor V Leiden, the G20210A mutation in the prothrombin gene, and protein S or protein C deficiency.

Anti-phospholipid syndrome: This autoimmune syndrome is characterised by the presence of antibodies directed against phospholipids, components of cell membranes. These antibodies increase the risk of thrombosis.

6. Deep vein thrombosis (DVT): Symptoms and specific features

DVT is the formation of a blood clot in a deep vein, most often in the lower limbs. In pregnant women, DVT can develop insidiously, making it difficult to diagnose.

Clinical signs :

Calf pain and tenderness: Pain is often the first symptom, described as a feeling of heaviness, cramp or tension in the calf. Palpation of the area may be painful.

Unilateral oedema of the lower limb: Oedema, or swelling, is a classic sign of DVT. It is important to compare the two legs to detect any difference in size.

Dilated superficial veins: Visible dilated superficial veins can be a sign of DVT, indicating obstruction of the deep venous system.

Positive Homans' sign: Dorsiflexion of the foot (bringing the foot towards the tibia) can trigger calf pain in DVT. This sign is not specific to DVT and may be present in other pathologies.

Erythema and local heat: The skin in the affected area may be red and warm to the touch, a sign of inflammation.

Specific features for pregnant women:

The symptoms of DVT may be masked by the physiological symptoms of pregnancy, such as leg oedema and fatigue.

DVT can develop in atypical veins, such as pelvic or ovarian veins, making diagnosis more complex.

7. Pulmonary Embolism (PE): A Vital Emergency

PE is a serious complication of DVT that occurs when a fragment of the clot breaks away and migrates to the lungs, obstructing one or more pulmonary arteries. PE is a medical emergency requiring immediate treatment.

Clinical signs :

Sudden onset of dyspnoea: Dyspnoea, or breathlessness, is the most common symptom and the most suggestive of PE. It is often sudden in onset and worsens with exertion.

Chest pain: Chest pain can be pleuritic (worsening on inspiration) or angina-like (constrictive, similar to heart pain).

Tachycardia: Increased heart rate is a physiological response to reduced blood oxygenation.

Hypotension: A drop in blood pressure can be a sign of shock, a serious complication of PE.

Syncope: loss of consciousness may occur in the event of massive PE, obstructing a large part of the pulmonary circulation.

Haemoptysis: Spitting up blood is a less frequent sign, but is still suggestive of PE.

Cyanosis: The bluish colouration of the skin and mucous membranes reflects a reduction in blood oxygenation.

8. Primary Prevention: Acting Upstream

Primary prevention aims to reduce the risk of VTE in pregnant women at risk. Mobilisation and mechanical measures are the cornerstones of this approach.

Early mobilisation after childbirth: Resuming walking and physical activity as soon as possible after giving birth promotes venous return and prevents blood stasis.

Compression stockings: Compression stockings exert graduated compression on the legs, improving venous return and reducing the risk of blood clots.

Low molecular weight heparin (LMWH) prophylaxis: In pregnant women at high risk of VTE, the prescription of LMWH prophylaxis is recommended to prevent clot formation.

9. Secondary Prevention: Avoiding Recurrences

Secondary prevention aims to prevent recurrences of VTE in women who have already had an episode. Prolonged anticoagulant treatment is the key to this approach.

Prolonged anticoagulant treatment: Women with a history of VTE require prolonged anticoagulant treatment, generally for 6 weeks to 3 months after delivery, and sometimes longer depending on the risk of recurrence.

10. Secondary prevention: Personalised follow-up

The duration of anticoagulant treatment and the choice of anticoagulant agent depend on a number of factors, including the type of VTE, the presence of thrombophilia and individual risk factors.

LMWH: LMWH are the treatment of choice during pregnancy and breastfeeding, as they do not cross the placental barrier or pass into breast milk.

Anti-vitamin K (AVK) : VKAs, like warfarin, are effective in preventing recurrences of VTE, but they cross the placental barrier and can cause congenital malformations. They are therefore contraindicated during pregnancy.

11. Treatment: Multidisciplinary Management

The treatment of VTE during pregnancy requires close collaboration between the midwife, obstetrician, haematologist and, if necessary, other specialists. The aim is to prevent the thrombus from spreading, encourage it to dissolve and prevent complications, while minimising the risks to the mother and foetus.

Curative-dose LMWH: In cases of DVT or PE, the initial treatment consists of curative-dose LMWH, adjusted according to the patient's weight.

Clinical and biological monitoring: Regular follow-up is necessary to monitor the efficacy of treatment and detect any adverse effects. This includes clinical assessment of symptoms, monitoring of anti-Xa levels (for LMWH), and platelet counts, as there is a risk of heparin-induced thrombocytopenia.

Treatment of the underlying cause: If an underlying cause of VTE is identified, such as thrombophilia, specific treatment may be required.

12. In depth : Dilemmas and Challenges

The management of VTE during pregnancy presents specific challenges.

Bleeding risk: Anticoagulants increase the risk of bleeding, which can be particularly worrying during childbirth. A careful assessment of the benefit-risk ratio is required.

Choice of delivery method : The mode of delivery depends on a number of factors, including the location and extent of the DVT, the type of anticoagulant used, and the presence of obstetric complications.

Breast-feeding and anticoagulants : Most LMWH are compatible with breast-feeding. However, VKAs are contraindicated during breast-feeding.

13. Conclusion: Vigilance and collaboration

VTE is a serious complication of pregnancy that requires constant vigilance and multidisciplinary care. Midwives play a crucial role in identifying women at risk, recognising clinical signs, implementing preventive measures and coordinating care with other healthcare professionals. Awareness of this condition and inter-professional collaboration are essential to ensure the safety and well-being of pregnant women and their babies.

14. Going further: Specialised aspects of MTE

To complete your understanding of VTE in pregnancy, it is useful to explore some more specialist aspects:

a. Thrombophilia and pregnancy :

Screening: Systematic screening for thrombophilia in all pregnant women is not recommended. However, targeted screening is recommended for women with specific risk factors, such as a personal or family history of VTE, repeated miscarriages or unexplained obstetric complications.

Management: The management of pregnant women with thrombophilia requires close collaboration between the obstetrician and haematologist. Preventive treatment with LMWH is often recommended during pregnancy and post-partum.

b. Anti-phospholipid syndrome and pregnancy :

Diagnosis: The diagnosis of anti-phospholipid syndrome is based on the presence of anti-phospholipid antibodies in the blood and a history of thrombosis or obstetric complications.

Management: Preventive treatment with LMWH and low-dose aspirin is generally recommended during pregnancy and the post-partum period.

c. MTE and Assisted Reproduction Techniques :

Increased risk: Women undergoing assisted reproductive technology (ART) have an increased risk of VTE, probably due to the hormonal treatments used and the risk factors underlying infertility.

Prevention: An assessment of the risk of MTE and the implementation of appropriate preventive measures are essential in pregnant women after TRA.

d. Psychological impact of ETD :

Anxiety and depression: The diagnosis of VTE during pregnancy can lead to significant anxiety and an increased risk of depression.

Psychological support: Adequate psychological support is essential to help women cope with the emotional impact of CWD.

e. Research and Development:

New anticoagulants: Research is underway to develop new, safer direct-acting oral anticoagulants (DAAs) during pregnancy.

Biomarkers: The search is on for more precise biomarkers to predict the risk of VTE and monitor the effectiveness of treatment.

15. Conclusion: Knowing, Acting, Supporting

VTE during pregnancy is a complex and evolving subject. As a midwife, your role is to acquire the knowledge needed to identify women at risk, recognise the clinical signs, implement preventive measures and collaborate effectively with other healthcare professionals to ensure optimal care. Your ability to support pregnant women with this condition, both physically and psychologically, is essential to ensuring a positive and reassuring pregnancy experience.

As a future midwife, you have the power to make a difference to the lives of women and their families. Invest in your training, keep up to date with the latest advances, and commit to providing quality care with compassion and expertise.

References :

1 American College of Obstetricians and Gynecologists. ACOG Practice Bulletin No. 196: Thromboembolism in pregnancy. Obstet Gynecol. 2018 May;131(5):e164-e179. (This bulletin provides comprehensive, up-to-date recommendations on the management of Thromboembolism in pregnancy based on the latest scientific evidence).

2 Royal College of Obstetricians and Gynaecologists. Green-top Guideline No. 37a: Reducing the risk of thrombosis and embolism during pregnancy and the puerperium. 2015. (This practical guide provides

detailed clinical guidelines for the prevention and treatment of VTE in pregnant and postpartum women).

3 James AH, Jamison MG, Brancazio LR, Myers ER. Venous thromboembolism during pregnancy and the postpartum period: incidence, risk factors, and mortality. Am J Obstet Gynecol. 2006 Apr;194(4):1311-5. (This research article examines the incidence, risk factors, and mortality associated with VTE during pregnancy and the postpartum period, providing important data for understanding this condition).

MCQS:

1. What are the three main physiological changes that increase the risk of VTE during pregnancy?

a) Increase in blood volume, reduction in blood pressure, increase in cardiac output

b) Hypercoagulability, venous stasis, endothelial lesions

c) Decreased haemoglobin level, increased white blood cell count, decreased platelet count

d) Increase in respiratory frequency, decrease in lung capacity, increase in oxygen consumption

e) Decreased renal function, increased urination, fluid retention

2. Which of the following is NOT considered a risk factor for VTE in pregnancy?

a) Personal history of TEN

b) Obesity

c) Multiple pregnancy

d) Blood group AB

e) Prolonged immobilisation

3. What is the main symptom of a pulmonary embolism?

a) Calf pain and swelling

b) Nausea and vomiting

c) Sudden onset of dyspnoea

d) Headaches and dizziness

e) Abdominal pain

4. What is the treatment of choice for the prevention of VTE in high-risk pregnant women?

a) Low-dose aspirin

b) Unfractionated heparin

c) Anti-vitamin K drugs (AVK)

d) Low molecular weight heparin (LMWH)

e) Iron supplementation

5. Why are anti-vitamin K (AVK) drugs contraindicated during pregnancy?

a) They are ineffective in preventing MTE.

b) They cross the placental barrier and can cause congenital malformations.

c) They increase the risk of arterial hypotension.

d) They interfere with the absorption of nutrients.

e) They cause frequent allergic reactions.

6. What type of healthcare professional specialises in the diagnosis and treatment of coagulation disorders such as thrombophilia?

a) Obstetrician

b) Paediatrician

c) Haematologist

d) Endocrinologist

e) Nephrologist

7. Why do women using assisted reproductive techniques (ART) have an increased risk of VTE?

a) Because of the increased risk of ectopic pregnancy.

b) Because of the hormonal treatments used and the risk factors underlying infertility.

c) Because of the increased risk of pre-eclampsia.

d) Because of the increased risk of premature delivery.

e) Because of the increased risk of congenital malformations.

8. What is one of the main challenges in the management of VTE during pregnancy?

a) The risk of adverse effects of anticoagulants on the foetus.

b) The difficulty in obtaining a precise diagnosis of TEN.

c) The high cost of anticoagulant treatments.

d) Lack of availability of MTE specialists.

e) Increasing resistance to anticoagulant treatments.

Answers:

1. b)
2. d)
3. c)
4. d)
5. b)
6. c)
7. b)
8. a)

Transfusion in obstetrics

Educational objectives :

1. Identify the main transfusion indications for different blood derivatives

2. List the main risks associated with blood transfusions.

3. Explain the rules for preventing transfusion accidents, the principles of blood product traceability and the haemovigilance system.

4. What immediate steps should be taken in the event of a poorly tolerated transfusion reaction?

1. Introduction :

Obstetric haemorrhage remains a major concern in maternal health, contributing significantly to maternal mortality and morbidity worldwide. Blood transfusion, when used judiciously and safely, becomes a vital tool for managing these critical situations and saving lives. This course explores in depth the complexities of blood transfusion in obstetrics, focusing on essential knowledge for midwives.

2. Lifesaving blood products (LBS): A detailed look

Red Blood Cell Concentrates (RBCs): Rich in haemoglobin, they are indicated to restore the blood's oxygen-carrying capacity in cases of severe anaemia or acute haemorrhage. Different formulas exist, such as leucocyte-reduced and irradiated RBCs, which are used according to the clinical context.

Fresh Frozen Plasma (FFP): Contains all the coagulation factors and is used to correct coagulopathies and prevent excessive bleeding. FFP can be used in emergency situations or in preparation for surgery.

Platelet concentrates (PCs): Essential for controlling bleeding due to thrombocytopenia or platelet dysfunction. PCs are often used in obstetrics in the context of massive post-partum haemorrhage.

Cryoprecipitate: Rich in fibrinogen, factor XIII and von Willebrand factor, it is used to treat haemorrhage associated with fibrinogen deficiency, such as in the case of disseminated intravascular coagulation (DIC).

3. Transfusion indications in obstetrics: a range of situations

Post-partum haemorrhage: transfusion of RGCs is the mainstay of treatment for post-partum haemorrhage, aimed at restoring blood volume and oxygen-carrying capacity. FFP and PCs may be necessary in cases of coagulopathy or thrombocytopenia.

Severe anaemia: When haemoglobin is less than 7 g/dL and affects the health of the mother or foetus, a transfusion of RGCs may be considered. The cause of the anaemia must be identified and treated.

Haemostasis disorders: transfusions of PFC, CP or cryoprecipitate are used to correct specific deficiencies in coagulation factors, platelets or fibrinogen.

Preparation for surgery: In the event of scheduled surgery and pre-existing anaemia or coagulation disorders, martial therapy or a transfusion of RGCs or FFPs may be necessary to optimise the patient's condition.

4. Pre-transfusion procedures: guaranteeing safety

ABO and Rhesus grouping: Essential for determining blood compatibility between donor and recipient and preventing haemolytic reactions.

Irregular Agglutinin Test (RAI): Detects the presence of antibodies directed against erythrocyte antigens other than the ABO and Rhesus antigens, making it possible to avoid delayed haemolytic transfusion reactions.

Compatibility test: A crucial step in confirming the compatibility between the donor's blood and that of the recipient, by carrying out a blood and/or serum test.

Blood typing: consists of separately ABO typing a drop of the patient's blood and a drop of blood from the transfusion bag.

Be careful, *the two drops of blood are never mixed* to test compatibility.

The serum test: consists of bringing the patient's **serum** into contact with a drop of blood from the transfusion bag.

Informed Consent: The patient must be informed of the risks and benefits of the transfusion, as well as the possible alternatives, before giving her consent.

5. Management of an Ill-Tolerated Transfusion: Immediate Reactivity

Stop transfusion immediately and call for help: The first step to take if a transfusion reaction is suspected.

Maintaining a patent venous line: Allows fluids and medication to be administered if necessary.

Monitoring vital parameters: Monitor blood pressure, pulse, respiratory rate and temperature for signs of haemodynamic instability or allergic reaction.

Blood samples: Blood samples are needed to analyse the causes of the transfusion reaction and identify any abnormalities.

Reporting the event: All transfusion accidents must be reported immediately, to protect both the patient and the medical and legal authorities.

Symptomatic treatment: Depending on the nature of the reaction, specific treatments may be administered, such as antihistamines for allergic reactions or diuretics for volume overload.

6. Transfusion Accidents: Understanding the Risks

Acute Haemolytic Reaction: A serious complication due to the destruction of transfused red blood cells by the recipient's antibodies. Symptoms include fever, chills, back pain, hypotension and haemoglobinuria. Immediate treatment is vital to prevent kidney failure and death.

Non-Haemolytic Febrile Reaction (NHFR): The most frequent reaction, characterised by fever and chills, generally harmless. It is often linked to the presence of antibodies directed against the donor's leukocytes.

Transfusion allergy: Allergic reactions to the donor's plasma proteins, manifested by urticaria, itching and even anaphylactic shock in severe cases.

Circulatory Volume Overload: An excess of transfused blood volume, which can lead to pulmonary oedema, especially in patients with a history of heart disease. Slow transfusion and careful monitoring of volume status are essential.

Transmission of infectious agents: Although the risk is low thanks to rigorous screening tests, the transmission of infectious diseases such as HIV, hepatitis B and C, and syphilis remains a concern.

7. Accidental Blood Exposure: Prevention and Management

Midwives are exposed to the risk of contact with contaminated blood when caring for patients.

Prevention: The use of personal protective equipment (PPE), such as gloves, masks and goggles, is essential to minimise the risk of exposure. Careful handling of needles and sharp objects is also crucial.

Management: In the event of accidental exposure, a specific protocol must be followed, including cleaning the exposed area, reporting the incident and assessing the risk of transmission of infectious agents. Post-exposure prophylaxis (PEP) may be necessary depending on the type of exposure and the infectious status of the source.

8. Conclusion: Committing to transfusion safety

Blood transfusion, although potentially life-saving, carries inherent risks. Midwives play a key role in promoting transfusion safety by ensuring that transfusions are appropriately indicated, that safety procedures are followed and that patients are informed of the risks and benefits. Ongoing vigilance, training and adherence to best practice are essential to optimise outcomes for pregnant women and their babies.

9. Exploring key concepts in greater depth

Haemovigilance: A system for monitoring adverse events related to blood transfusion, making it possible to identify risks and implement preventive measures.

Alternatives to Transfusion: Strategies to reduce the need for blood transfusions, such as active management of the third stage of labour, the use of haemostatic agents and autologous blood recovery techniques.

Transfusion ethics: Ethical issues surround blood transfusion, including informed consent, resource allocation and religious beliefs.

References :

1. Ministry of Solidarity and Health. Haemovigilance - Guide to good practice. 2019. (Provides information on the surveillance system for adverse events related to blood transfusion)

2. Collège National des Gynécologues Obstétriciens Français (CNGOF). Post-partum haemorrhage - What to do. Recommendations for clinical practice. 2014. (Provides recommendations on the management of post-partum haemorrhage, including the use of blood transfusion)

3. Agence nationale de sécurité du médicament et des produits de santé (ANSM). Good blood transfusion practices. 2017. (Details the good practices to be followed during blood transfusions to ensure patient safety).

Questions :

Q1: The main indication for blood transfusion in obstetrics is..:

a) Moderate anaemia

b) Post-partum haemorrhage

c) Preparing for a scheduled caesarean section

d) Minor haemostasis disorders

e) Pregnancy-induced hypertension

Q2: The labile blood product used to increase the oxygen-carrying capacity of the blood is :

a) Fresh frozen plasma (FFP)

b) Platelet concentrates (PCs)

c) Red blood cell concentrates (RBCs)

d) Cryoprecipitate

e) Immunoglobulins

Q3: Irregular agglutinin tests (RAI) are used to :

a) Determining ABO and Rhesus blood groups

b) Testing for the presence of anti-erythrocyte antibodies

c) Measuring haemoglobin levels

d) Assessing platelet function

e) Identifying transmissible infectious agents

Q4: A clinical sign suggestive of an acute haemolytic reaction is :

a) A skin rash

b) Lower back pain

c) A dry cough

d) Chills without fever

e) Nausea and vomiting

Q5: The first action to take in the event of a suspected transfusion reaction is :

a) Administer an antihistamine

b) Increasing the transfusion rate

c) Stop the transfusion immediately

d) Taking a blood sample

e) Contact the doctor in charge

Q6: The most frequent transfusion reaction, generally benign, is :

a) Acute haemolytic reaction

b) Non-haemolytic febrile reaction

c) Transfusion allergy

d) Circulatory volume overload

e) Transmission of infectious agents

Q7: The personal protective equipment (PPE) used when handling blood includes :

a) Gloves, mask and goggles
b) A sterile gown and cap
c) Safety shoes and apron
d) A mask and cap
e) A full-body suit

Q8: The haemovigilance system makes it possible to :
a) Improving blood product stock management
b) Monitoring adverse transfusion reactions
c) Training nursing staff in transfusion techniques
d) Promoting blood donation
e) Funding blood transfusion research

Q9: An example of an alternative to blood transfusion is :
a) Oxygen administration
b) Active management of the third stage of labour
c) Transfusion of fresh frozen plasma
d) Fetal heart rate monitoring
e) Oral administration of iron

Q10: Informed consent for a blood transfusion involves :
a) Obtaining the spouse's agreement
b) Informing the patient of the risks and benefits
c) Signing a standard form
d) Consulting an ethics committee
e) Carrying out additional tests

MCQ answers :

1. b, 2. c, 3. b, 4. b, 5. c, 6. b, 7. a, 8. b, 9. b, 10. B

Shock in obstetrics

Learning objectives :

1. Distinguish between the four types of obstetric shock (haemorrhagic, anaphylactic, septic and cardiogenic).

2. Recognise the clinical signs and pathophysiological mechanisms of each type of shock.

3. Implementing the initial therapeutic management of states of shock.

4. Organising care with the medical team in an emergency situation.

1. Introduction

Obstetric shock is a life-threatening emergency, affecting both mother and foetus. It is characterised by acute circulatory failure that deprives vital organs of oxygen and nutrients. Rapid and effective management is crucial to minimise complications and improve prognosis. This course aims to provide you with the knowledge you need to identify, understand and manage the different types of shock encountered in obstetric practice.

2. Definitions

Shock is a complex clinical syndrome resulting from a mismatch between tissue oxygen requirements and actual supply. This tissue hypoperfusion leads to cellular and organ metabolic disturbances, which can progress to multiple organ failure and death. There are four types of shock, depending on their origin:

Haemorrhagic shock: Caused by massive blood loss, this is the most common form of haemorrhage in obstetrics, and occurs in cases of delivery haemorrhage, uterine rupture, etc.

Anaphylactic shock: Sudden generalised life-threatening allergic reaction caused by exposure to an allergen (drugs, latex, etc.).

Septic shock: organ dysfunction resulting from a disproportionate systemic inflammatory response to an infection, often of bacterial origin.

Cardiogenic shock: acute cardiac dysfunction preventing the heart from delivering sufficient blood flow to meet the body's needs.

3. Diagnostic approach

When faced with a patient presenting with signs of shock, a rigorous and rapid diagnostic approach is essential:

Anamnesis and clinical examination: Take a medical history and describe the circumstances in which the shock occurred, and look for signs of shock (tachycardia, hypotension, polypnoea, oliguria, altered consciousness) and signs specific to each type of shock.

Haemodynamic monitoring: Measure blood pressure, heart rate, oxygen saturation and diuresis to assess cardiovascular function and tissue perfusion.

Additional tests: Biological tests (CBC, ionogram, lactate, etc.) and medical imaging (ultrasound, X-ray, etc.) to confirm the diagnosis, identify the cause of the shock and assess organ damage.

4. Etiopathogenesis

Each type of shock has specific pathophysiological mechanisms, but all converge on tissue hypoperfusion:

Haemorrhagic shock: Blood loss reduces circulating blood volume, leading to a drop in cardiac output and organ hypoperfusion, activating compensatory mechanisms that may prove insufficient if blood loss persists.

Anaphylactic shock: The massive release of vasoactive mediators (histamine, etc.) causes systemic vasodilation, increased capillary permeability and fluid leakage into the tissues, reducing effective blood volume and arterial pressure.

Septic shock: The systemic inflammatory response to infection results in vasodilation, increased capillary permeability, coagulation disorders and myocardial dysfunction, leading to tissue hypoperfusion and multiple organ failure.

Cardiogenic shock: Cardiac dysfunction reduces cardiac output and arterial pressure, compromising organ perfusion and activating compensatory mechanisms that may prove ineffective if cardiac function does not improve.

5. Haemorrhagic shock

a. Definition

Haemorrhagic shock, the most common form of haemorrhage in obstetrics, is the result of acute and significant blood loss that can occur at various stages of pregnancy and the post-partum period (childbirth, placenta previa, premature detachment of the placenta, uterine rupture, ectopic pregnancy, etc.).

b. Pathophysiology

Blood loss reduces circulating blood volume, activating compensatory mechanisms (tachycardia, peripheral vasoconstriction) to maintain blood pressure. If blood loss persists, these mechanisms become insufficient, leading to a drop in cardiac output, tissue hypoperfusion and metabolic acidosis.

c. Clinical examination

Signs of shock: Pallor, tachycardia, hypotension, polypnoea, oliguria, mottling, agitation, confusion.

Specific signs: Profuse metrorrhagia, hypotonic uterus, abdominal pain.

d. What to do

Alerting the medical and anaesthetic team: Multidisciplinary management is essential for a rapid, coordinated response.

High-flow oxygen therapy: Ensuring optimal oxygenation of tissues.

Large-bore peripheral venous access and vascular filling: Restore circulating blood volume by administering crystalloids and/or colloids.

Blood transfusion if necessary: To correct the anaemia and restore the oxygen-carrying capacity of the blood.

Treatment of the cause of the haemorrhage: Identify and treat the source of the blood loss (uterotonic drugs, suture, embolisation, surgery).

6. Anaphylactic shock

a. Definition

Anaphylactic shock is a severe allergic reaction that sets in suddenly and can be fatal. It occurs following exposure to an allergen, triggering a massive release of vasoactive mediators. Common causes in obstetrics include drugs (antibiotics, anaesthetics), latex, blood products and hymenoptera venoms.

b. Pathophysiology

Exposure to the allergen triggers the massive release of histamine and other vasoactive mediators by mast cells and basophils. These mediators cause systemic vasodilation, increased capillary permeability, bronchospasm and smooth muscle contraction, leading to a sudden drop in blood pressure and tissue hypoperfusion.

c. Clinical examination

Signs of shock: Hypotension, tachycardia, polypnoea.

Skin signs: Urticaria, pruritus, flush, angioedema.

Respiratory signs: Bronchospasm, dyspnoea, stridor.

Digestive signs: Nausea, vomiting, abdominal pain, diarrhoea.

d. What to do

Alerting the medical and anaesthetic team: Immediate care is crucial.

Stop administering the suspected allergen: Identify and stop exposure to the allergen.

High-flow oxygen therapy: Maintain adequate oxygenation.

Intramuscular or intravenous adrenaline: Counteracts the effects of vasoactive mediators and restores blood pressure.

Vascular filling with crystalloids: Increase circulating blood volume and improve tissue perfusion.

Corticosteroids and antihistamines: Reduce inflammation and allergic symptoms.

7. Septic shock

a. Definition

Septic shock is a serious medical emergency, characterised by life-threatening organ dysfunction resulting from the body's inadequate response to infection. In obstetrics, surgical site infections, urinary tract infections, chorioamniotitis and post-partum endometritis are frequent causes of septic shock.

b. Pathophysiology

Infection triggers an excessive systemic inflammatory response, with the release of pro-inflammatory mediators (cytokines, etc.). These mediators cause vasodilatation, increased capillary permeability, coagulation disorders and myocardial dysfunction, leading to tissue hypoperfusion and multi-visceral failure.

c. Clinical examination

Signs of shock: Hypotension, tachycardia, polypnoea, oliguria, altered consciousness.

Signs of infection: fever, chills, abdominal pain, foul-smelling vaginal discharge.

d. What to do

Alert the medical and anaesthetic team: multidisciplinary management is necessary.

High-flow oxygen therapy: Ensuring adequate oxygenation of tissues.

Bacteriological samples: to identify the germ responsible and adapt antibiotic therapy.

Intravenous broad-spectrum antibiotics: Treat the infection rapidly.

Vascular filling with crystalloids: Improving tissue perfusion.

Treatment of the source of the infection: abscess drainage, surgery if necessary.

8. Cardiogenic shock

a. Definition

Cardiogenic shock is a medical emergency resulting from acute cardiac dysfunction, preventing the heart from maintaining adequate blood flow to meet the body's needs. In obstetrics, it can be caused by cardiomyopathy, pulmonary embolism, aortic dissection or a complication of anaesthesia.

b. Pathophysiology

Cardiac dysfunction leads to a reduction in cardiac output and arterial pressure, compromising organ perfusion. Compensatory mechanisms, such as tachycardia and peripheral vasoconstriction, are activated, but become insufficient if cardiac function does not improve.

c. Clinical examination

Signs of shock: Hypotension, tachycardia, polypnoea, oliguria, altered consciousness.

Cardiac signs: Heart murmur, galloping noise, acute pulmonary oedema, chest pain.

d. What to do

Alert the medical and anaesthetic team: specialised care is required.

High-flow oxygen therapy: Ensuring optimal oxygenation of tissues.

Haemodynamic monitoring: To assess cardiac function and tissue perfusion.

Treatment of the cause of cardiac dysfunction: inotropic drugs, diuretics, vasodilators, etc.

Circulatory assistance if necessary: Consider circulatory assistance devices in the event of severe heart failure.

9. Conclusion

Obstetric shock is a life-threatening emergency requiring rapid recognition, immediate treatment and close collaboration between healthcare professionals. Midwives play a crucial role in the early detection of signs of shock, the implementation of initial therapeutic measures and alerting the medical team. A good knowledge of the different types of shock and how to manage them is essential to ensure the safety of mother and child.

10. Exploring key concepts in greater depth

Lactates: Blood lactate levels are an important marker of the severity of shock and tissue hypoperfusion. In hypoxic conditions, cellular metabolism switches to anaerobic conditions, increasing lactate production.

SOFA score: Sequential Organ Failure Assessment (SOFA) is a score used to assess organ failure and the severity of septic shock. It takes into account parameters from different systems (respiratory, cardiovascular, hepatic, renal, neurological and haematological) and enables the patient's progress to be monitored.

Cardiac output: Cardiac output is the volume of blood pumped by the heart per minute. It is an important indicator of cardiac function and tissue perfusion. Low cardiac output can lead to organ hypoperfusion and shock.

Mean arterial pressure (MAP): MAP is a measure of the mean blood pressure in the arteries during a cardiac cycle. It is an important indicator of organ perfusion. A low MAP may indicate shock and tissue hypoperfusion.

References :

1. James AH, Steer PJ. Obstetric Hemorrhage: A Comprehensive Guide to Evaluation and Management. 2nd ed Wiley-Blackwell; 2012.

2. Joint Task Force on Practice Parameters; American Academy of Allergy, Asthma & Immunology; American College of Allergy, Asthma and Immunology; Joint Council of Allergy, Asthma and Immunology. Anaphylaxis: A Practice Parameter Update 2020. J Allergy Clin Immunol. 2020 Oct;146(4):823-881.

3. Evans L, Rhodes A, Alhazzani W, Antonelli M, Coopersmith CM, French C, et al. Surviving Sepsis Campaign: International Guidelines for Management of Sepsis and Septic Shock 2021. Crit Care Med. 2021 Oct 1;49(10):e1063-e1143.**

4. McDonagh TA, Metra M, Adamo M, Gardner RS, Baumbach A, Böhm M, et al. 2021 ESC Guidelines for the diagnosis and treatment of acute and chronic heart failure. Eur Heart J. 2021 Nov 1;42(36):3599-3726.

Questions :

1. What is the most common type of shock in obstetrics?

A. Anaphylactic shock

B. Cardiogenic shock

C. Haemorrhagic shock

D. Septic shock

E. Neurogenic shock

Answer: C.

2. Which of the following statements about anaphylactic shock is FALSE?

A. It is triggered by exposure to an allergen.

B. It is characterised by systemic vasoconstriction.

C. It can cause bronchospasm and respiratory distress.

D. Adrenaline is the first-line treatment.

E. Corticosteroids and antihistamines are used as adjuvant treatment.

Answer: B.

3. What is the main biological marker of tissue hypoperfusion in shock?

A. Haemoglobin

B. Leukocytes

C. Inserts

D. Lactates

E. Creatinine

Answer: D.

4. Which of the following is NOT a clinical sign of shock?

A. Tachycardia

B. Bradycardia

C. Hypotension

D. Polypnoea

E. Oliguria

Answer: B.

5. The SOFA score is used to evaluate :

A. The severity of the haemorrhage.

B. The severity of the anaphylactic reaction.

C. Organ failure in septic shock.

D. Cardiac function in cardiogenic shock.

E. The risk of respiratory distress.

Answer: C.

Anaesthesia and Analgesia in Obstetrics

Educational objectives :

1. Describe the different types of anaesthesia used during labour.

2. Explain the potential maternal-foetal consequences of these anaesthetic techniques.

3. Describe the steps involved in providing epidural analgesia for childbirth.

4. Name the important parameters to be monitored during epidural analgesia for childbirth.

Part 1: Anaesthesia and Analgesia in Labour

1. Introduction :

A patient in early labour who is suffering from algae has the right to receive a modern and effective analgesia technique, without obstetric, maternal or neonatal consequences.

To provide analgesia for labour or anaesthesia for childbirth, you need to be familiar with the physiological changes in pregnant women and the maternal-foetal consequences of these techniques.

2. Epidemiology :

Recently, there has been an increase in the caesarean section rate. With increasing use of spinal anaesthesia and less recourse to general anaesthesia.

For vaginal deliveries, analgesia for labour is now widespread (epidural for 63% of deliveries).

3. Pregnancy-related physiological changes :

a. Changes to the nervous system :

Requirements for inhaled anaesthetic agents (IAAs) are reduced by around 30% during pregnancy. Progesterone and beta endorphins, levels of which increase considerably during pregnancy, appear to be involved in these changes in sensitivity to anaesthetic products. Indeed, the pain threshold is increased during pregnancy. The need for local anaesthetics is also reduced by 20-30%, not only by the reduction in volume of the epidural space due to the turgidity of the epidural venous plexuses, but also by an increase in the sensitivity of nerve fibres to local anaesthetics. The sensitivity of peripheral nerve fibres to local anaesthetics is also increased.

b. Musculoskeletal changes :

Increased lordosis with narrow intervertebral spaces can make axial blocks difficult.

In pregnant women, there is a greater risk of cranial extension of the spinal block in a strict dorsal decubitus position, which is why it is advisable to place the patient in a slight left diversion to free up venous return, with a slight elevation of the head.

c. Pharmacodynamic changes :

High circulating progesterone levels lead to increased sensitivity to local anaesthetics (LA) during epidural anaesthesia. The concentration and volumes must therefore be reduced: for example, 0.125% bupivacaine.

The almost systematic addition of liposoluble morphines reduces the minimum concentration of local anaesthetic.

The myocardial toxicity of bupivacaine is higher during pregnancy.

4. Types of anaesthesia and maternal-foetal consequences :

A patient in early labour and suffering from pain has the right to receive a modern and effective analgesia technique, without obstetric, maternal or neonatal consequences:

- If entry into labour and cervix dilated by 4 cm => epidural analgesia (APD)
- If cervix dilated to 10cm and head engaged => rachi anaesthesia (RA) end of labour
- If HTAG + vaginal route accepted => APD

- If leaky valve insufficiency is not advanced + no contraindication to LRA => APD

Light" DPAs: (local protocol must be followed)

- Lower concentration of bupivacaine or ropivacaine
- The addition of a fat-soluble morphine (sufentanil or fentanyl) reduces the dose of local anaesthetic.

With "light" APD, there was a significant reduction in the undesirable effects of high-dose APD. Light" APD is the best technique for controlling the pain of labour, and is just as effective as "high dose" APD. It does not alter the duration of the first part of labour and has no deleterious effect on the newborn. It significantly lengthens the second stage of labour (by 15 minutes on average), increases the use and consumption of oxytocics and increases the use of instrumental extractions (not significant in the latest meta-analyses);

An intrarachid passage :

In the event of APD, the appearance of rapid and marked hypotension, breathing difficulties or the early appearance of significant motor block, and more often than not abnormalities in the foetal heart rate (FHR) are the signs that should prompt us to stop the infusion of anaesthetic product.

=> Immediate resuscitation + removal of the epidural catheter + placement of an epidural in another space with more cautious doses.

5. Analgesia in labour: the main principles

a. Peri-medullary anaesthesia and analgesia

The puncture is most often performed at L3-L4. The advantage of a low-level puncture (L2 to L5) is that it limits the risk of direct trauma to the spinal cord, as in the vast majority of cases the marrow terminates at L1. The use of a test dose is therefore still under discussion. The first injection is better tolerated from a haemodynamic point of view if it is performed in the lateral decubitus position rather than in the sitting position. The impact of the epidural is greater in the sitting position. Epidural anaesthesia is not always possible. The first contraindication is refusal on the parturient's part. There are other contraindications.

b. Possible complications:

The complications to be feared are the risk of the formation of a compressive peri-medullary haematoma (haemostasis and/or coagulation disorders, aspirin and anticoagulant medication), the risk of developing a peri-medullary infection (local or generalised infection) and the risk of potentially significant and deleterious haemodynamic repercussions linked to the vasoplegia induced by the epidural (haemorrhage and/or uncontrolled hypovolaemia, severe cardiac pathology) as well as other risks such as certain specific neurological pathologies, and above all post dura mater breach headaches.

c. Contraindications:

Perimedullary ALR is contraindicated if :

- Patient refusal;
- Abnormalities of haemostasis and/or coagulation ;
- Systemic or localised (lumbar) infections ;
- Specific neurological pathologies;

- Unstable hemodynamic state ;
- Severe maternal haemorrhage ;
- Very severe valve disease (calcific aortic stenosis)

d. Monitoring :

Clinical monitoring must ensure maternal and foetal safety.

It is essential to monitor BP every 5 minutes for 30 minutes after injecting the product, and to continuously monitor the FHR.

Secondly, it is important to ensure that the analgesia is effective, by aiming for the disappearance of the pain associated with the contractions with even the smallest dose of local anaesthetic, and to check for the presence of an adequate sensory block by testing for a sensation of heat and/or tingling in both feet, vasodilation of the veins of the feet, and by checking the level of the sensory block to ensure that it goes all the way back to D10 during the dilation phase (hot/cold, prick/touch).

e. Pre-anaesthetic consultation :

The anaesthetic consultation with a biological check-up (at the end of pregnancy) to screen for these possible contraindications, to organise with the obstetric team the management of antiaggregant or anticoagulant treatment (therapeutic window for low molecular weight heparins [LMWH] and to offer patients alternatives to DPA), to stop LMWH at least 12 hours before DPA in the case of prophylactic treatment, and at least 24 hours if the treatment is curative and to stop calciparin at least 8 hours before DPA in the case of curative treatment.

f. End of labour anaesthesia

If there are no contraindications and if the local conditions are favourable for accepting the vaginal route immediately, we opt for an AR: hyperbaric Bupivacaine 5 mg + sufenta 2.5µg.

g. Parenteral analgesia

All parenterally administered morphine crosses the placental barrier and is likely to modify the variability of the FHR. Pethidine is currently being abandoned. Remifentanil may have a place in rare situations, but beware of respiratory distress in the newborn.

6. Conclusion

As with all anaesthesia, a preanaesthetic consultation with a targeted assessment and verification of contraindications to LRA is necessary for epidural analgesia or end-of-labour anaesthesia.

It is advisable to reduce the concentration of the local anaesthetic and add a fat-soluble morphine, and to carefully monitor the tolerance and efficacy of the procedure.

Part 2: Anaesthesia for Caesarean section

1. Introduction :

To ensure an uneventful caesarean delivery, you need to be fully aware of the physiological changes associated with pregnancy, prepare the woman for the operation and the anaesthetic, choose the right anaesthetic technique and apply an early rehabilitation protocol.

2. Pre-anaesthetic consultation for pregnant women :

To prepare the parturient for peripartum anaesthesia, her anaesthetic consultation should be scheduled early, to assess her haemodynamically, respiratorily, haematologically and hormonally, especially in view of the physiological changes associated with pregnancy that must be taken into account, to request a minimum work-up (GS, CBC), and to request other targeted examinations in a targeted manner.

All in all, we need to look for pathologies associated with pregnancy (HTAG, gestational diabetes...) and stabilise chronic diseases and manage treatments.

3. Degree of urgency of the different indications for caesarean section :

Caesarean section is indicated in extreme emergencies, within 5 minutes, if there is cord prolapse, retroplacental haematoma, permanent foetal bradycardia or maternal cardio respiratory arrest.

Emergency indications lasting 10 to 15 minutes are: a pathological cardiofœtal rhythm, obstructed labour, abnormally inserted haemorrhagic placenta, scar disunion or worsening of a maternal pathology.

Indications for an emergency delayed by 20 to 30 minutes are: cervical dystocia, failure of labour to progress, pathological cardiofetal rhythm, non-haemorrhagic placental insertion anomaly, or maternal and/or foetal pathology with labour in progress.

4. Choice of anaesthetic technique for Caesarean section :

Full-term pregnant women are at risk of difficult intubation and are also considered to have a full stomach. The anaesthetic technique of choice for pregnant women is therefore rachi anaesthesia.

However, if there is a contraindication to rachi-anaesthesia or in the case of an emergency caesarean section, general anaesthesia is the solution, with precautions to manage the airways and maintain haemodynamics.

If an epidural catheter has already been inserted, extending the anaesthetic through the catheter is the appropriate technique.

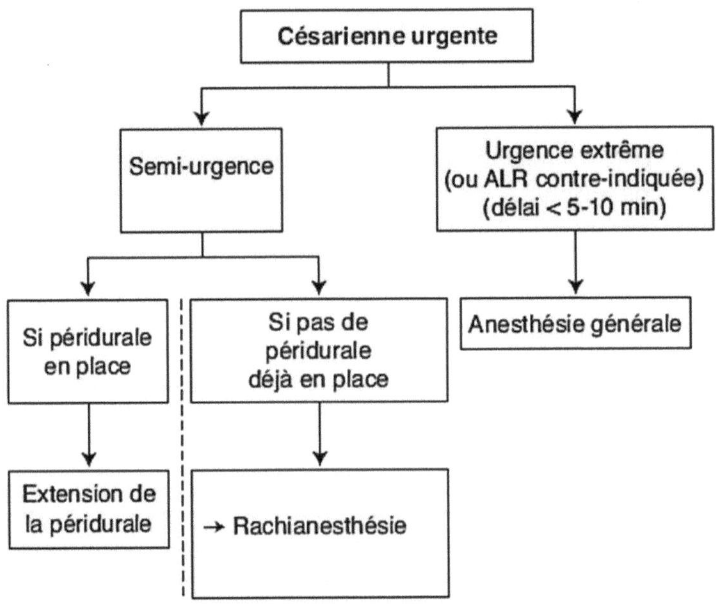

Figure : Choice of anaesthetic technique according to the degree of urgency of the caesarean section

(https://sofia.medicalistes.fr/spip/IMG/pdf/anesthesie_pour_cesarienne.pdf)

Type d'anesthésie	Avantages	Risques ou Inconvénients
Anesthésie générale (AG)	Perte de conscience Contrôle de la ventilation Contrôle hémodynamique Levée d'analgésie progressive Rapidité d'installation Protection cérébrale du nouveau-né	Difficulté d'intubation Inhalation de liquide gastrique Allergies Complications de la ventilation Analgésie postopératoire systémique Nouveau-né endormi Inhalation amniotique Pic hypertensif à l'intubation
Anesthésie locorégionale (ALR)	Pas de perte de conscience Accueil de l'enfant Pas d'intubation Analgésie postopératoire Sécurité du réveil Éveil de l'enfant nouveau-né	Délai d'installation variable Difficulté technique du geste Levée d'analgésie brutale Hypotension Complications infectieuses Complications neurologiques

Table: Advantages and disadvantages of anaesthetic techniques depending on the indication for caesarean section

a. Spinal anaesthesia :

Contraindications:

Peri-medullary ALR is contraindicated if :

- Patient refusal;
- Abnormalities of haemostasis and/or coagulation ;
- Systemic or localised (lumbar) infections ;
- Specific neurological pathologies;
- Unstable hemodynamic state ;

- Severe maternal haemorrhage ;
- Very severe valve disease (calcific aortic stenosis)

Protocol :

This involves mixing hyperbaric Bupivacaine 10 mg with Sufentanil 5µg and intrathecal Morphine 100µg, using a 25 G pencil point needle, targeting the L3-L4 space, to achieve a sensory level below D4 and a Bromage score below M2.

Complications :

The complications to be feared are the risk of the formation of a compressive peri-medullary haematoma (haemostasis and/or coagulation disorders, aspirin and anticoagulant medication), the risk of developing a peri-medullary infection (local or generalised infection) and the risk of potentially significant and deleterious haemodynamic repercussions linked to the vasoplegia induced by the epidural (haemorrhage and/or uncontrolled hypovolaemia, severe cardiac pathology) as well as other risks such as certain specific neurological pathologies, and above all post dura mater breach headaches.

If the dura mater is breached, there will be headaches that are aggravated by standing up, calmed by decubitus, painkillers, hydration and coffee. Prevention involves a single injection using a 25-gauge pencil-point needle. Treatment consists of hyperhydration, analgesics and coffee. If there is no improvement, a Blood patch should be made.

b. General anaesthesia :

The indications for general anaesthesia in pregnant women are becoming increasingly limited, because the risk of difficult intubation and the risk of inhalation (during induction or extubation) is greater in this population, from 16 weeks' gestation onwards, and especially as the woman approaches term and goes into labour.

This general anaesthetic must be given after preparation of the difficult intubation tray, which is a source of functional mucus aspiration. In the context of a caesarean section, induction should only take place if all the surgical equipment is ready and the obstetrician is also ready, scalpel in hand. Long-acting morphine drugs (Fentanyl, sufentanil, etc.)

should be administered after foetal extraction to avoid transplacental passage and possible neonatal respiratory distress.

Induction should be rapid. It should be preceded by pre-oxygenation (8 vital capacities on O2 10l/minutes), then started by the administration of propofol followed by succinylcholine, and after 60 seconds orotracheal intubation is performed.

The administration of morphine during induction is only indicated in pregnant women if there is a history of gravid hypertension with high blood pressure, or a history of valvulopathy. In these cases, remifentanil should be preferred, as it has a short duration of action and is therefore associated with a lower risk of neonatal respiratory distress.

c. Postpartum monitoring and post-caesarean section rehabilitation:

In the post-partum period, strict monitoring of the following parameters (blood pressure, pulse, uterine globe and appearance of bleeding) prevents 60% of cases of post-partum haemorrhage (PPH), especially in the presence of risk factors for PPH.

The next step is to ensure fluid intake until solids can be taken orally, to keep the bladder catheter in place until 8 hours post-operatively, to ensure appropriate multimodal analgesia (paracetamol, NSAIDs, morphine), to ensure preventive anticoagulation with anti-thrombotic stockings and to encourage the mother to get up early and walk around to avoid complications associated with prolonged decubitus.

References:

1. Chestnut's Obstetric Anaesthesia: Principles and Practice (6th ed.) - A comprehensive book covering all aspects of obstetric anaesthesia.

2. Practice Guidelines for Obstetric Anesthesia - An updated report from the American Society of Anesthesiologists and the Society for Obstetric Anesthesia and Perinatology, providing evidence-based clinical recommendations.

3. UpToDate - A regularly updated online resource offering comprehensive, evidence-based information on a variety of medical topics, including obstetric anaesthesia.

4. Bengayed k, Khalifa C, Maghrebi H. Post-Caesarean Rehabilitation: Evaluation Of Practices. (2024) Journal of Health and Rehabilitation Research, 4(1), 1214-1218. https://doi.org/10.61919/jhrr.v4i1.439

Effects of anaesthetic drugs on pregnant women

Educational objectives :

1. Explain the main physiological changes induced by pregnancy.

2. To identify the implications of these changes for the pharmacokinetics and pharmacodynamics of anaesthetic drugs.

1. Introduction

Pregnancy is a unique physiological state that generates numerous physiological adaptations in women. These adaptations are designed to support the development of the foetus and prepare the mother's body for childbirth. However, they also modify the pregnant woman's response to anaesthetic drugs, requiring a thorough understanding and adaptation of anaesthetic techniques to ensure the safety of both mother and foetus.

2. Haemodynamic changes and anaesthetic implications

Pregnancy induces significant haemodynamic changes, including a 30-50% increase in cardiac output, a 40-45% increase in blood volume and a decrease in systemic vascular resistance. These changes make pregnant women more sensitive to the hypotensive effects of anaesthetics, increasing the risk of maternal and foetal complications.

Compression of the inferior vena cava by the pregnant uterus, particularly in the supine position, can lead to a cave syndrome. This syndrome is characterised by maternal hypotension, reduced venous return to the heart and foetal hypoxia.

Implications:

Close monitoring of blood pressure: Allows accurate assessment of blood pressure and early detection of potential hypotension, particularly in patients at risk of cave syndrome.

Adequate hydration: Preventive volume expansion helps to compensate for vasodilatation and maintain adequate blood pressure.

Use of vasopressors: Vasopressors such as phenylephrine may be required to maintain blood pressure and uteroplacental perfusion.

Left lateral decubitus position: This position relieves compression of the inferior vena cava, improves venous return and prevents cava syndrome.

3. Respiratory changes and anaesthetic implications

Increased oxygen consumption, CO2 production and reduced functional residual capacity make pregnant women more susceptible to hypoxia and hypercapnia. Oedema of the airway mucosa, combined with increased vascularisation, can make tracheal intubation more difficult.

Implications:

Pre-oxygenation oxygenation: administering 100% oxygen before anaesthetic induction increases the oxygen reserve and prolongs apnoea time in complete safety.

Close monitoring of oxygen saturation: Enables early detection of hypoxaemia and rapid intervention.

Anticipating a difficult intubation: preparing an alternative intubation plan and using appropriate instruments.

Prevention of aspiration of gastric contents: Gastric emptying is slowed during pregnancy, increasing the risk of aspiration. Prophylactic measures, such as the administration of antacids and antiemetics, are essential.

4. Haematological changes and anaesthetic implications

The physiological hypercoagulability of pregnancy, combined with the compression of pelvic veins by the gravid uterus, increases the risk of deep vein thrombosis and pulmonary embolism. The physiological anaemia of pregnancy, due to a disproportionate increase in plasma volume in relation to the mass of red blood cells, may require particular attention.

Implications:

Antithrombotic prophylaxis: Compression stockings and/or low molecular weight heparin may be prescribed for patients at risk of venous thromboembolism.

Blood transfusion: If the anaemia is severe, a blood transfusion may be necessary to optimise oxygen transport.

5. Other physiological changes and anaesthetic implications

Pregnancy also modifies hepatic metabolism and renal clearance, influencing drug pharmacokinetics. The upward displacement of the diaphragm reduces lung capacity, and the relaxation of the ligaments increases the risk of joint trauma during manipulation.

3. Exploring key concepts in greater depth

Pharmacokinetics and pharmacodynamics: Pregnancy modifies the absorption, distribution, metabolism and elimination of drugs. Understanding these changes means that doses and administration schedules can be adapted to achieve the desired effects while minimising the risks to the mother and foetus.

Transplacental passage of medicines: Medicines administered to the mother can cross the placenta and reach the foetus, potentially affecting its development and health. The choice of drugs should take into account their potential for transplacental passage and their effects on the foetus.

Anaesthesia techniques: General anaesthesia, locoregional anaesthesia (epidural, spinal anaesthesia) and obstetric analgesia are the main techniques used in obstetrics. The choice of technique depends on the operation envisaged, the patient's preferences, her medical history and the health of the foetus.

4. Conclusion

Anaesthesia for pregnant women requires an individualised approach and specific expertise. Understanding the physiological changes, knowing the pharmacokinetic and pharmacodynamic implications, and mastering the appropriate anaesthesia techniques are essential to ensure optimal care and guarantee the safety of both mother and foetus.

References

1. Chestnut, D. H., Wong, C. A., Tsen, L. C., Kee, W. D., Beilin, Y., Mhyre, J. M., Polley, L. S. (2014). Chestnut's Obstetric Anesthesia: Principles and Practice. Elsevier Health Sciences.

2. Datta, S. (2015). Anaesthesia for Cesarean Section. Springer.

3. Hawkins, J. L., Koonin, L. M., Palmer, S. K., & Gibbs, C. P. (2011). Anesthesia-related deaths during obstetric delivery in the United States, 1979-2002. Anesthesiology, 115(1), 27-34.

4. Lyons, G., & Macdonald, R. (2009). Physiology in childbearing with anatomy and related biosciences. Elsevier Health Sciences.

Questions

1. Explain why pregnant women are more sensitive to the hypotensive effects of anaesthetics.

Answer: Pregnant women have reduced systemic vascular resistance and increased cardiac output, making them more susceptible to the hypotensive effects of anaesthetics.

2. Describe the main measures for preventing cave syndrome in pregnant women undergoing anaesthesia.

Answer: Measures to prevent cava syndrome include positioning the patient in a left lateral decubitus position, adequate hydration and the use of vasopressors.

3. What impact does pregnancy have on drug pharmacokinetics?

Answer: Pregnancy alters the absorption, distribution, metabolism and elimination of drugs, which may mean that doses and administration schedules need to be adapted.

Newborn resuscitation in the delivery room

Theoretical objectives :

1. Explain foetal respiratory physiology

2. Describe foetal and neonatal blood circulation

3. Describe the list of equipment for resuscitating newborn babies in the delivery room.

4. Describe the principles of neonatal resuscitation

1. Introduction :

Among newborns, 10% require assistance in the delivery room, 3% require positive pressure ventilation and 0.1% require intensive resuscitation with chest compressions and adrenaline to complete their transition to life outside the womb.

Priority should be given to respiratory resuscitation and normothermia should be maintained at between 36.5°C and 37.5°C during resuscitation, whatever the term.

There were some minor differences between the American and European recommendations concerning the length of cord clamping delay (30 sec or 1 min), the number of initial ventilations and the emergency route.

The principles of neonatal resuscitation are based on the physiological changes that occur during the transition from intrauterine to extrauterine life.

If there are any risk factors, in utero transfer should be considered.

We must emphasise the value of simulation-based teaching techniques.

2. Physiological reminder :

a. During intrauterine life :

Exchanges between foetus and mother are by diffusion. Fetal haemoglobin HbF is very sensitive to oxygen (O2) and the haemoglobin level is 17 g/100 ml at the end of pregnancy. The foetal lung has no respiratory function. Pulmonary resistance is high. Pneumocytes are immersed in alveolar fluid.

During intrauterine life :

The umbilical vein (VO) brings nutrient- and O2-enriched blood from the placenta.

O2 saturation is around 80%. Oxygenated blood from the placenta reaches the IVC via the duct of Arantius and then the DO.

The latter also receives venous return from the SCV.

In the foetus, the 2 circulations are in parallel and the pressures in the right cavities are high.

There are 3 shunts between the 2 circuits:

- The Arantius canal (between the VO and VCI)
- The foramen ovale (FO) between the 2 atria. 40% of oxygenated blood from the placenta passes from the OD to the OG and then to the LV and the aorta. 60% of oxygenated blood passes into the VD and the pulmonary artery,
- The ductus arteriosus, at the level of the aortic isthmus, allows blood from the PA to communicate with blood from the aorta coming from the LV.

The opening of the ductus arteriosus is always located downstream of the start of the brachiocephalic trunk, enabling the territory of supraductal vascularisation (coronary arteries, brain, right upper limb) to be determined.

This is why, in the first few minutes of life, we insist on measuring O2 saturation using pulsed oximetry on the right hand.

Some of the blood from the descending aorta returns to the placenta via the 2 umbilical arteries.

O2 saturation is between 50 and 60%.

b. Transitional circulation

At the moment of birth: the onset of breathing and cord clamping (clamping should be delayed by at least 30 seconds to 1 minute) modify the shunts, gradually leading to the definitive post-natal circulation.

The first cries and efficient breathing help to build up a functional residual capacity (FRC). O2 from the ambient air reaches the alveoli. The FRC is built up during the first respiratory cycles in parallel with the resorption of alveolar fluid (activation of sodium pumps by endogenous catecholamines in early labour).

Initially, compliance is low and significant respiratory effort is required (high pressures or prolonged inspiratory time), before breathing becomes effortless.

Surfactant forms a surface-active film on the surface of the alveoli and stabilises the CRF.

Mediators are released: endogenous nitric oxide (NO) and the postaglandin PGE2. Pulmonary vascular resistance falls and pulmonary blood flow increases.

Functional pulmonary circulation induces an increase in pulmonary venous return and therefore an increase in pressure in the OG.

The pressure in the OG becomes greater than that in the OD, and the foramen ovale closes.

Clamping the cord increases systemic vascular resistance. Performed after the first respiratory cycles, it allows better adaptation to initial variations in ventricular volume.

Pressures rise in the left cavities and fall in the right cavities. The result is a post-natal circulation in series with high systemic pressure and low pulmonary pressure. Each ventricle will differentiate with an increase in the contractile mass of the LV (multiplied by 3 during the first 3 weeks of life).

The ductus arteriosus will shunt bidirectionally:

o left-right shunt (AO to AP) with increasingly oxygenated blood leading to functional closure by progressive vasoconstriction and then anatomical closure

o right-left shunt of desaturated blood, which decreases as the AO/AP pressure gradient increases.

Preductal blood is not contaminated by this D-G shunt. This is why the pulsed oximetry (SpO2) sensor on the right hand reflects the oxygenation of the blood vascularising the brain.

In a newborn who adapts normally to air, SpO2 values follow the Dawson curve, rising from 60% in the first minute of life to 90% at 10 minutes.

Triggering efficient breathing is the key to successful adaptation to life outside the womb.

3. Equipment in the delivery room :

To avoid wasting unnecessary time, the equipment is always operational and checked before each birth.

The recommended room temperature is at least 25°C, and 26°C in the case of an expected premature birth of less than 32 weeks' gestation.

The resuscitation table with stopwatch is checked: suction set at between 100 and 150 cm H2O, 6 to 12 suction probes, thermal probe, multiparameter monitor (HR, SpO2, BP), air/O2 mixer, manual insufflator with pressure control, T-piece at best.

If there is no T-piece, the self-inflating balloon for term or near-term newborns has a volume of 450-500 ml.

The ventilation frequency is 40-50/min with a 3-stroke rhythm:

Res (insuflation)----pi----rer

Intubation equipment must be checked.

Tracheal intubation :

o Mask ventilation is ineffective or prolonged

- When chest compressions are performed, in order to optimise ventilation
- Immediately in case of diaphragmatic hernia

In the case of mask ventilation or after intubation, a 6-gauge gastric tube is inserted in premature babies or an 8-gauge tube in full-term babies, to empty the air from the stomach and allow better thoracic ampliation.

The drugs used for resuscitation are adrenaline diluted 1:10, preferably administered by the venous route, via an umbilical venous catheter, rather than by the intra-tracheal route, which is still possible.

9 ‰ saline as a filling solution and glucose solutions.

Blood glucose levels must be measured, and blood gas, haemoglobin and lactate analyses taken.

The following requirements must be met:

- Speed and coordination without rushing (phases A-B-C-D in order)

- Normothermia between 36.5°C and 37.5°C

- Asepsis (hydroalcoholic solution, gloves, gown, cap and mask if invasive procedures)

The 2 main evaluation criteria are :

- Breathing
- Heart rate best assessed by ECG

ECG monitoring has been indicated since 2015. Pulse oximetry underestimates heart rate in the first few minutes of life during transitional circulation.

The Apgar score no longer leads to resuscitation.

Reconstituted after resuscitation, it is used to assess the speed of recovery and has prognostic value.

Resuscitation is guided by the heart rate and its evolution.

Oxygenation is assessed by preductal SpO_2.

The first 2 people in charge.

A (airway) :

- Stopwatch

- Dry and stimulate the baby,

- Ensure the airways are free: neutral position of the newborn, clear the airways (2/3 anterior to the mouth and 0.5 to 1 cm from the entrance to the nostrils without crossing the choanae) if necessary, with a vacuum of 100 to 150 cmH2O.

- Aspiration that is too deep triggers vagal bradycardia in the first ten minutes.

- The bonnet is put on at the same time.

- The premature baby < 32 SA during phase A is wrapped in a polyethylene bag without drying it.

B (breathing) :

- If HR < 100/min: positive pressure ventilation is initiated before the end of the 1st minute, regardless of the appearance of the fluid.

- Using a mask and balloon or, better still, a T-piece as described in the equipment section.

- The only contraindication is diaphragmatic hernia, which requires intubation from the outset.

- Assess ventilation efficiency after 30 sec.

If the heart rate does not rise and the chest does not rise, check :

o F: Leaks? "check equipment, reposition mask

o O: Obstruction? "Aspiration, opening of the mouth; in the event of meconium fluid, tracheo-aspiration.

o P: Insufficient pressure? "Pressures are increased (underlying respiratory disease).

o The frequency is 40 to 60 c/min.

- Insufflation pressures are 20 to 25 cmH2O in a full-term infant and 15 to 20 cmH2O in a premature infant, to be adapted according to the lift of the thorax.

- The PEEP is 4 to 5 cmH2O for term newborns and 5-6 cmH2O for premature babies.

- FiO2 is started at 21% (advantage of the mixer) and then according to the supraductal SpO2.

- The operators look at the chest, the pressure needle and the monitor (ECG, SpO2).

- If the HR > 100 b/min after 30 seconds of ventilation, we adapt to the resumption of spontaneous ventilation.

- The intubation attempt should be limited to 20-30 seconds. If this fails, the child is taken back by mask and the oxygen titrated.

C: to ensure an efficient circulatory minimum.

- Assess heart rate after 30 sec of effective ventilation.

- If initial ventilation is ineffective, after correction of the PFO, the patient is restarted with 30 sec of ventilation.

- If HR < 60 b/min: start CTs alternating with ventilation: 3 CTs for ventilation (120/min).

(The CTs: while packing the chest, the 2 thumbs meet at the lower 1/3 of the sternum, 1 cm below the nipple line. This technique has been judged preferable to the 2-finger technique).

- As soon as CT is used, increase FiO2 to 100%.

- Intubation can optimise ventilation if it has not been performed beforehand.

- As soon as a TC is required, a 3rd person is called in.

D (drugs) = medicines :

After 30 sec of CT, we assess whether the HR is:

•60/min, the CTs are stopped and ventilation continues.

•< 60/min, adrenaline is indicated, preferably IV via KTVO at a dose of 10 to 30 µg/kg.

A 4th person is needed to help install the KTVO.

If resuscitation is ineffective, we must always consider :

- Malposition or displacement of the tracheal tube

- Hypovolaemia

- Pneumothorax

- A pulmonary malformation

- Diaphragmatic hernia

- Heart disease

E: stands for environment and family.

- Any resuscitation of a newborn child is anxiety-provoking for the parents.

- Give them clear, factual information.

- We advise you to be careful.

- If the child is transferred, pass on the information given to the parents to the transport team and the receiving department.

Encouraging contact between children and their parents (touch, photos, etc.)

When should resuscitation be stopped? :

- Stop resuscitation in a still lifeless NN (no pulse, no respiratory movement) after 10 min of continuous and adapted resuscitation efforts.

- In the case of HR < 60/min at birth and remaining so after 10 to 15 min of continuous, well-performed resuscitation, there is insufficient evidence of outcome to guide the decision to discontinue or continue resuscitation.

- Practices are at the discretion of each country.

- Nevertheless, we must take into account: the cause of the cardiorespiratory arrest, the gestational age, the severity of any malformation, the possibility of reversibility of the situation, the degree of morbidity and sequelae agreed by the parents during the immediate antenatal or postnatal interview.

- In most cases, the newborn is admitted in a serious condition to the neonatal intensive care unit, where his or her case is discussed by the entire team.

4. Post-resuscitation care :

The NN is reviewed in its entirety, with reassessment and continued stabilisation of the major vital functions.

The Apgar score is reconstructed.

If the NN has regained respiratory autonomy, we look for signs of respiratory distress: polypnoea, Silvermann score.

In the event of insufficient oxygenation and/or signs of respiratory distress, CPAP is applied with a T-piece, followed by a NIV interface on the ventilator, with FiO2 titrated according to SpO2 figures.

If the NN is dependent on mask ventilation, intubation is performed.

The place where the NN is received will depend on its recovery and the type of maternity hospital.

A precise record of the resuscitation is drawn up, including the times.

Birth in meconium fluid :

If the child born with meconium fluid is adapting well, only a VAS deobstruction is performed.

Close respiratory monitoring (clinical, SpO2) and neurological monitoring are carried out.

The recommendations only advocate anticipation, with the presence of a person competent in the intubation of NN.

5. Conclusion:

-NN resuscitation follows a precise A-B-C-D-E algorithm.

-Ventilation is essential.

Delayed clamping of the cord, monitoring techniques, the importance of maintaining normothermia during resuscitation, the adverse effects of hyperoxia, the end of intra-tracheal suctioning in the event of a birth in meconium fluid, except in the event of an obstacle, the end of prophylactic intubation of extremely premature babies, therapeutic hypothermia in the event of Hypoxic-Ischaemic Encephalopathy.

-Repeated procedural, simulation and team training sessions for birth room staff are necessary.

6. References

Resuscitation of the newborn in the delivery room; Essentiel© 2017 conference, Sfar, Paris

MCQS :

Question 1: What proportion of newborns require respiratory assistance in the delivery room?

a) 1%

b) 3%

c) 10%

d) 20%

e) 50%

Question 2: What is the main role of pulmonary surfactant?

a) Increasing pulmonary vascular resistance

b) Reducing lung compliance

c) Stabilising functional residual capacity

d) Facilitating the passage of blood from the DO to the OG

e) Allow closure of the ductus arteriosus

Question 3: Where should the pulse oximetry sensor be placed to reflect cerebral blood oxygenation?

a) Right foot

b) Left hand

c) Right hand

d) Right ear

e) Left ear

Question 4: When should chest compressions be started?

a) HR < 100/min

b) HR < 80/min

c) HR < 60/min

d) SpO2 < 80

e) SpO2 <70

Question 5: What is the main route of administration of adrenaline?

a) Intraosseous

b) Intramuscular

c) Intra-tracheal

d) Subcutaneous

e) Venous

Question 6: What is the main indication for immediate intubation in neonates?

a) Meconium fluid

b) Prematurity

c) Diaphragmatic hernia

d) Bradycardia

e) Hypotonia

Question 7: When should resuscitation be stopped?

a) HR < 60/min after 5 minutes of resuscitation

b) Absence of spontaneous breathing after 5 minutes of ventilation

c) SpO2 < 80% after 10 minutes of oxygen therapy

d) Absence of pulse and respiration after 10 minutes of resuscitation

e) Persistent hypotonia after 15 minutes of resuscitation

Question 8: What is the benefit of delayed cord clamping?

a) Promoting closure of the ductus arteriosus

b) To enable better adaptation to initial variations in ventricular volume

c) Increasing lung compliance

d) Reducing pulmonary vascular resistance

e) Facilitating the resorption of alveolar fluid

Question 9: What guides neonatal resuscitation?

a) Apgar score

b) Preductal SpO2

c) Heart rate

d) Respiratory rate

e) Blood pressure

Answers:

1-c ; 2-c ; 3-a ; 4-c ; 5-e ; 6-c ; 7-d ; 8-b ; 9-c

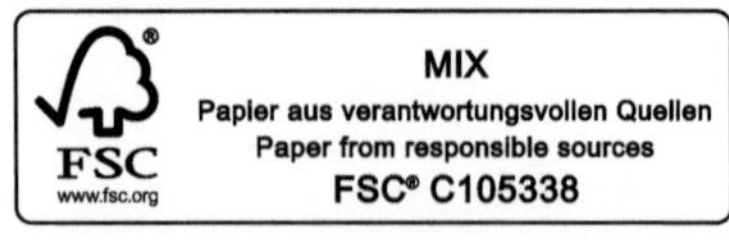

Printed by Books on Demand GmbH, Norderstedt / Germany